THE GALLBLADDER DIET
BIBLE

Controlling Gallbladder Symptoms Via Dietary Modifications & The Significance Of A Gallbladder-Friendly Diet

CRUE GAGE

Table of Contents

Introductory

The gallbladder plays a crucial role in digestion, particularly in the breakdown and absorption of fats. Here are its primary functions:

• **Storage**: The gallbladder stores bile, a digestive fluid produced by the liver. Bile is essential for emulsifying fats, breaking them down into smaller particles that enzymes can digest more effectively.

• **Release of Bile**: When fatty foods enter the small intestine, the gallbladder contracts and releases bile into the duodenum (the first part of the small intestine). This bile helps in the digestion and absorption of fats and fat-soluble vitamins (like A, D, E, and K).

• **Bile Composition**: Bile consists of bile salts, cholesterol, bilirubin, and water.

Bile salts aid in fat digestion and absorption by breaking down fat globules into smaller droplets, making it easier for pancreatic enzymes to access them.

• **Regulation**: The release of bile from the gallbladder is triggered by hormonal signals, especially after the ingestion of fatty foods. The bile duct transports bile from the liver and gallbladder to the small intestine.

• **Biliary System**: The gallbladder is part of the biliary system, which includes the liver, bile ducts, and pancreas. This system works together to facilitate the digestion and absorption of nutrients, especially fats.

Issues like gallstones or inflammation can affect the gallbladder's function, leading to discomfort and complications.

Common Gallbladder Problems

Common gallbladder problems include:

• **Gallstones**: These are the most frequent issues, where solid particles form in the gallbladder from bile components. Gallstones can vary in size and number and may cause pain if they block the bile ducts.

• **Cholecystitis**: This refers to inflammation of the gallbladder, often due to gallstones blocking the bile ducts or causing irritation. It can lead to severe pain, fever, and sometimes infection.

• **Biliary Colic**: This is intense pain caused by a gallstone obstructing the cystic duct or bile ducts, typically occurring after meals high in fat.

• **Choledocholithiasis**: Gallstones that move into the bile ducts can cause blockages, leading to symptoms such as jaundice (yellowing of the skin and eyes), abdominal pain, and nausea.

• **Cholangitis**: This is an infection in the bile ducts, usually caused by bacteria ascending from the intestines into the bile ducts, often due to a blockage from gallstones.

• **Gallbladder Polyps**: These are growths on the inner surface of the gallbladder, often benign but sometimes requiring monitoring or treatment.

• **Dysfunctional Gallbladder**: Sometimes the gallbladder may not empty properly, causing symptoms similar to gallstones or cholecystitis without actual stones.

Treatment for gallbladder problems can range from dietary changes and medications to surgical removal of the gallbladder (cholecystectomy), especially in cases of recurrent or severe issues like gallstones and cholecystitis.

CHAPTER ONE
Foods To Include And Avoid

When managing gallbladder issues or aiming to prevent them, dietary choices can play a crucial role. Here's a general guideline for foods to include and avoid:

Foods to Include:

- **High-Fiber Foods**: Whole grains, fruits, and vegetables can help regulate digestion and prevent constipation, which may worsen gallbladder symptoms.

- **Healthy Fats**: Choose sources of healthy fats such as olive oil, avocados, and fatty fish (like salmon and trout), which are easier to digest compared to saturated fats.

- **Lean Proteins**: Opt for lean meats like chicken, turkey, and fish. Plant-based proteins like beans and legumes are also good choices.

- **Low-Fat Dairy**: Choose low-fat or fat-free dairy products to reduce the load on your gallbladder.

- **Plenty of Water**: Staying hydrated is important for overall digestive health.

- **Moderate Caffeine**: While moderate amounts of caffeine (like in coffee and tea) are generally fine, excessive caffeine intake may worsen symptoms for some individuals.

Foods to Avoid or Limit:

- **High-Fat Foods**: Fried foods, fatty meats, full-fat dairy products, and rich desserts can trigger gallbladder symptoms or worsen existing conditions.

- **Processed Foods**: Avoid processed foods high in trans fats and unhealthy oils, as these can be hard to digest.

- **Spicy Foods**: Spicy foods can sometimes irritate the digestive system and exacerbate symptoms.

- **High-Sugar Foods**: Sugary foods and beverages can contribute to weight gain and may exacerbate gallbladder issues.

- **Alcohol**: Limit alcohol consumption, as it can affect liver function and bile production.

- **Gas-Producing Foods**: Some people find that certain foods like onions, cabbage, and beans can cause gas and discomfort.

Always consult with a healthcare provider or a registered dietitian for personalized dietary recommendations based on your specific health needs and any existing gallbladder issues.

Macronutrient Balance (Carbohydrates, Proteins, Fats)

The macronutrient balance, particularly for individuals with gallbladder issues or those looking to support gallbladder health, should be balanced and tailored to individual needs. Here's a general guideline:

Carbohydrates:

• Carbohydrates should primarily come from whole grains, fruits, and vegetables. These sources provide fiber, which aids in digestion and helps regulate bowel movements. Avoid or minimize refined carbohydrates and sugary foods, as they can contribute to weight gain and may aggravate symptoms.

Proteins:

• Choose lean sources of protein such as poultry (without skin), fish, beans, legumes, and low-fat dairy products. These proteins are easier to digest and are generally better tolerated by individuals with gallbladder issues compared to fatty cuts of meat or high-fat dairy products.

Fats:

• Focus on consuming healthy fats such as monounsaturated fats found in olive oil, avocados, and nuts, as well as omega-3 fatty acids from fatty fish like salmon and trout. These fats are beneficial for overall health and easier on the digestive system compared to saturated and trans fats found in fried foods, fatty meats, and processed snacks.

Balance:

A balanced approach typically includes:

- **Carbohydrates**: About 45-65% of your total daily calories.

- **Proteins**: About 10-35% of your total daily calories.

- **Fats**: About 20-35% of your total daily calories, with an emphasis on healthy fats.

Adjustments may be necessary based on individual tolerances and health conditions. Monitoring how your body responds to different macronutrient ratios can help you determine the best balance for managing gallbladder health effectively. Always consult with a healthcare provider or dietitian for personalized advice.

Importance Of Fiber And Hydration

Fiber and hydration play crucial roles in maintaining overall digestive health, including supporting gallbladder function. Here's why each is important:

Fiber:

• **Digestive Regularity**: Fiber adds bulk to stool, which helps promote regular bowel movements. This is important because constipation can contribute to the formation of gallstones and exacerbate symptoms of gallbladder issues.

• **Nutrient Absorption**: Soluble fiber, found in foods like oats, beans, and fruits, can help regulate blood sugar levels and improve nutrient absorption, which is beneficial for overall health.

• **Weight Management**: High-fiber foods tend to be filling and can help control appetite, which may support weight management. Maintaining a healthy weight is important for reducing the risk of gallstones and other gallbladder problems.

• **Gut Microbiome**: Fiber serves as a prebiotic, nourishing beneficial bacteria in the gut. A healthy gut microbiome is linked to improved digestion and overall health.

Hydration:

• **Bile Production**: Staying hydrated is essential for the production of bile, which is stored in the gallbladder and aids in the digestion and absorption of fats. Insufficient hydration can lead to thicker bile, potentially contributing to the formation of gallstones.

• **Digestive Health**: Water helps keep the digestive system functioning smoothly by aiding in the breakdown and absorption of nutrients. It also helps prevent constipation, which, as mentioned, is beneficial for gallbladder health.

• **Overall Health**: Proper hydration supports many bodily functions, including circulation, temperature regulation, and nutrient transport. It also helps flush toxins from the body, supporting overall health and well-being.

Recommendations:

• **Fiber Intake**: Aim for a variety of high-fiber foods, including fruits, vegetables, whole grains, legumes, and nuts. The recommended daily intake varies but generally ranges from 25-38 grams per day depending on age and gender.

- **Hydration**: Drink plenty of water throughout the day. The amount needed varies depending on factors like age, activity level, and climate, but a general guideline is about 8 cups (2 liters) of water per day.

By ensuring adequate fiber intake and staying well-hydrated, you can support your digestive system, promote gallbladder health, and contribute to overall wellness.

CHAPTER TWO
Sample Meal Plans For Different Dietary Needs

Here are sample meal plans tailored for different dietary needs, focusing on supporting gallbladder health by emphasizing fiber-rich foods, lean proteins, and healthy fats. These plans provide a balanced macronutrient profile and include foods that are generally well-tolerated by individuals with gallbladder issues.

Sample Meal Plan: Balanced Diet

Breakfast:

- Scrambled eggs with spinach and tomatoes
- Whole grain toast
- Fresh fruit (e.g., berries or apple slices)

Lunch:

- Grilled chicken salad with mixed greens, cucumber, bell peppers, and a vinaigrette dressing (made with olive oil)
- Whole grain roll or crackers

Afternoon Snack:

- Greek yogurt with a handful of nuts (e.g., almonds or walnuts)
- Carrot sticks or cucumber slices

Dinner:

- Baked salmon with quinoa and steamed broccoli
- Mixed green salad with avocado and a lemon-olive oil dressing

Evening Snack (if needed):

- Sliced apple with almond butter

Sample Meal Plan: Low-Fat Diet

Breakfast:

- Oatmeal topped with sliced banana and a drizzle of honey
- Low-fat milk or almond milk

Lunch:

- Turkey and vegetable wrap with whole grain tortilla
- Mixed greens salad with a light vinaigrette dressing

Afternoon Snack:

- Low-fat cottage cheese with pineapple chunks

Dinner:

- Grilled chicken breast with brown rice and steamed asparagus

- Steamed carrots

Evening Snack (if needed):

- Air-popped popcorn
- Sample Meal Plan: Vegetarian/Vegan

Breakfast:

- Smoothie made with spinach, banana, almond milk, and chia seeds
- Whole grain toast with avocado

Lunch:

- Quinoa salad with black beans, corn, cherry tomatoes, and a lime-cilantro dressing

Afternoon Snack:

- Hummus with raw vegetable sticks (e.g., carrots, bell peppers)

Dinner:

- Stir-fried tofu with mixed vegetables (e.g., broccoli, bell peppers, snap peas) and brown rice

Evening Snack (if needed):

- Mixed nuts and dried fruit

Tips for All Plans:

- **Hydration**: Drink plenty of water throughout the day.
- **Portion Control**: Pay attention to portion sizes to avoid overeating, which can stress the digestive system.

- **Avoid Trigger Foods**: Adjust these plans to avoid specific foods that may trigger symptoms for you personally.

If you have specific dietary restrictions or medical conditions, consult with a healthcare provider or registered dietitian for personalized advice. These sample meal plans provide a framework for building balanced, nutritious meals that support gallbladder health while accommodating different dietary preferences and needs.

Tips For Preparing Gallbladder-Friendly Meals

Preparing gallbladder-friendly meals involves making choices that promote digestion and reduce the risk of discomfort. Here are some tips to help you prepare meals that support gallbladder health:

• Opt for lean meats such as chicken, turkey, and fish. Remove skin and visible fat before cooking to reduce the load on your digestive system.

• Grill, bake, steam, or poach foods instead of frying them. This reduces the amount of added fats and makes meals easier to digest.

• Include plenty of fruits, vegetables, whole grains, beans, and legumes in your meals. Fiber aids digestion and helps regulate bowel movements, reducing the risk of constipation.

• Minimize consumption of foods high in saturated fats (like fatty cuts of meat, full-fat dairy) and avoid trans fats (found in processed and fried foods). These fats can be difficult to digest and may exacerbate gallbladder symptoms.

• Include sources of healthy fats such as olive oil, avocados, nuts, and seeds. These fats are easier on the digestive system and provide essential nutrients.

• Be mindful of portion sizes to avoid overeating, which can stress the digestive system and potentially trigger symptoms.

• Some people find that spicy foods can irritate the digestive system. If you're sensitive to spicy foods, consider minimizing or avoiding them.

• Drink plenty of water throughout the day to help maintain healthy bile production and support overall digestive function.

• Plan meals ahead of time to ensure they're balanced and include a variety of nutrient-rich foods. This can help you avoid last-minute unhealthy choices.

• Pay attention to how your body reacts to different foods. Keep a food diary if needed to identify trigger foods or patterns that worsen symptoms.

By following these tips, you can create meals that are gentle on your digestive system and supportive of gallbladder health. If you have specific dietary concerns or conditions, consulting with a healthcare provider or registered dietitian can provide personalized guidance.

CHAPTER THREE
Breakfast Recipes

Here are some gallbladder-friendly breakfast recipes that are nutritious, easy to prepare, and gentle on the digestive system:

1. Oatmeal with Berries and Almonds

Ingredients:

- 1/2 cup rolled oats
- 1 cup water or milk (such as almond milk)
- Handful of fresh berries (e.g., strawberries, blueberries)
- 1 tablespoon sliced almonds
- 1 teaspoon honey or maple syrup (optional)

Instructions:

- In a saucepan, bring water or milk to a boil.
- Stir in rolled oats and reduce heat to medium-low. Cook, stirring occasionally, until oats are tender and most of the liquid is absorbed (about 5-7 minutes).
- Remove from heat and transfer oatmeal to a bowl.
- Top with fresh berries, sliced almonds, and a drizzle of honey or maple syrup if desired.
- Enjoy warm.

2. Greek Yogurt Parfait with Fruit and Granola:

Ingredients:

- 1/2 cup plain Greek yogurt

- 1/2 cup fresh fruit (e.g., sliced banana, berries)
- 1/4 cup granola (choose a low-fat and low-sugar option)

Instructions:

- In a serving glass or bowl, layer Greek yogurt, fresh fruit, and granola.
- Repeat layers as desired.
- Serve immediately.

<u>3. Spinach and Feta Omelette:</u>

Ingredients:

- 2 eggs
- Handful of fresh spinach leaves
- 1-2 tablespoons crumbled feta cheese
- Salt and pepper to taste
- 1 teaspoon olive oil

Instructions:

- In a bowl, whisk together eggs with salt and pepper.
- Heat olive oil in a non-stick skillet over medium heat.
- Add spinach leaves to the skillet and sauté until wilted (about 1-2 minutes).
- Pour whisked eggs over the spinach, tilting the skillet to spread evenly.
- Cook until eggs are set and edges are golden brown, about 2-3 minutes.
- Sprinkle crumbled feta cheese over one half of the omelette.
- Fold the omelette in half and cook for another minute until cheese melts.
- Slide onto a plate and serve hot.

4. Smoothie with Spinach, Banana, and Almond Milk:

Ingredients:

- 1 cup fresh spinach leaves
- 1 ripe banana
- 1 cup almond milk (or any milk of your choice)
- 1 tablespoon almond butter (optional)
- Ice cubes (optional)

Instructions:

- Combine spinach, banana, almond milk, and almond butter (if using) in a blender.
- Blend until smooth and creamy.
- Add ice cubes if desired for a chilled smoothie.

- Pour into a glass and serve immediately.

Tips:

- **Variations**: Feel free to customize these recipes with your favorite fruits, nuts, or seeds.
- **Portion Control**: Pay attention to portion sizes, especially if you have specific dietary needs or goals.
- **Hydration**: Enjoy these meals with a glass of water to stay hydrated throughout the day.

These breakfast recipes provide a good balance of nutrients while being gentle on the digestive system, making them suitable for supporting gallbladder health.

Lunch Recipes

Here are some gallbladder-friendly lunch recipes that are nutritious, easy to prepare, and focus on lean proteins, healthy fats, and high-fiber ingredients:

1. Grilled Chicken and Quinoa Salad:

Ingredients:

- 1 boneless, skinless chicken breast
- 1/2 cup quinoa
- Mixed greens (e.g., spinach, arugula)
- Cherry tomatoes, halved
- Cucumber, sliced
- Red onion, thinly sliced
- Olive oil and balsamic vinegar for dressing
- Salt and pepper to taste

Instructions:

- Cook quinoa according to package instructions and set aside.
- Season chicken breast with salt and pepper, then grill until cooked through (about 4-5 minutes per side). Let it rest for a few minutes before slicing.
- In a large bowl, combine mixed greens, cherry tomatoes, cucumber, and red onion.
- Add cooked quinoa and sliced grilled chicken on top.
- Drizzle with olive oil and balsamic vinegar.
- Toss gently to combine and serve immediately.

2. Turkey and Avocado Wrap:

Ingredients:

- Whole grain tortilla wrap
- Sliced deli turkey (low-fat, nitrate-free)
- Avocado slices
- Baby spinach leaves
- Sliced bell peppers (optional)
- Hummus or mustard (optional)

Instructions:

- Lay the whole grain tortilla wrap flat on a clean surface.
- Spread a thin layer of hummus or mustard (if using) over the tortilla.
- Layer with sliced turkey, avocado slices, baby spinach, and sliced bell peppers.

- Roll the tortilla tightly and slice in half.
- Serve immediately or wrap tightly in foil for later.

3. Quinoa-Stuffed Bell Peppers:

Ingredients:

- Bell peppers (any color), halved and seeded
- 1 cup quinoa, cooked
- Black beans, drained and rinsed
- Corn kernels (fresh or frozen)
- Diced tomatoes (canned or fresh)
- Shredded low-fat cheese (optional)
- Fresh cilantro, chopped
- Salt and pepper to taste

Instructions:

- Preheat oven to 375°F (190°C).

- In a large bowl, mix cooked quinoa, black beans, corn, diced tomatoes, and fresh cilantro. Season with salt and pepper to taste.

- Stuff each bell pepper half with the quinoa mixture.

- Place stuffed bell peppers on a baking sheet lined with parchment paper.

- Bake for 25-30 minutes, or until peppers are tender and filling is heated through.

- If using cheese, sprinkle shredded cheese on top of stuffed peppers during the last 5 minutes of baking.

- Remove from oven and let cool slightly before serving.

4. Salmon and Asparagus Foil Packets:

Ingredients:

- Salmon fillet (skinless)
- Asparagus spears, trimmed
- Lemon slices
- Fresh dill, chopped
- Olive oil
- Salt and pepper to taste

Instructions:

- Preheat oven to 400°F (200°C).
- Cut a large piece of aluminum foil. Place salmon fillet in the center of the foil.
- Arrange asparagus spears around the salmon.
- Drizzle olive oil over salmon and asparagus. Season with salt, pepper, and chopped dill.

- Place lemon slices on top of the salmon.

- Fold the edges of the foil to create a sealed packet.

- Bake in the oven for 15-20 minutes, or until salmon is cooked through and asparagus is tender.

- Carefully open the foil packet and transfer salmon and asparagus to a plate.

- Serve hot, optionally with a side of quinoa or brown rice.

<u>Tips:</u>

- **Preparation**: These recipes can often be prepared ahead of time and stored for easy lunches throughout the week.

- **Customization**: Feel free to adjust ingredients based on personal preferences and dietary needs.

- **Portion Sizes**: Be mindful of portion sizes to ensure balanced nutrition and avoid overeating.

These lunch recipes provide a variety of flavors and textures while supporting gallbladder health through nutritious ingredients and healthy cooking methods.

Here are some gallbladder-friendly dinner recipes that focus on lean proteins, healthy fats, and high-fiber ingredients to support digestion and overall health:

1. Baked Lemon Herb Chicken with Quinoa and Steamed Broccoli:

Ingredients:

- 2 boneless, skinless chicken breasts
- Juice of 1 lemon
- 2 tablespoons olive oil
- 2 cloves garlic, minced
- 1 teaspoon dried thyme
- 1 teaspoon dried rosemary
- Salt and pepper to taste
- 1 cup quinoa, cooked
- Steamed broccoli florets

Instructions:

- Preheat oven to 400°F (200°C).

- In a small bowl, whisk together lemon juice, olive oil, minced garlic, dried thyme, dried rosemary, salt, and pepper.

- Place chicken breasts in a baking dish and pour the lemon herb marinade over them, ensuring they are evenly coated.

- Bake for 20-25 minutes, or until chicken is cooked through and juices run clear.

- While chicken is baking, prepare quinoa according to package instructions and steam broccoli florets.

- Serve baked lemon herb chicken with a side of quinoa and steamed broccoli.

<u>**2. Turkey and Vegetable Stir-Fry:**</u>

Ingredients:

- 1 lb ground turkey
- 2 cups mixed vegetables (e.g., bell peppers, snap peas, carrots)
- 1 tablespoon olive oil
- 2 cloves garlic, minced
- 1 tablespoon low-sodium soy sauce or tamari
- 1 teaspoon sesame oil
- Cooked brown rice or quinoa for serving

Instructions:

- Heat olive oil in a large skillet or wok over medium-high heat.
- Add minced garlic and sauté for 1 minute until fragrant.

- Add ground turkey and cook until browned and cooked through, breaking it up with a spoon as it cooks.

- Add mixed vegetables to the skillet and stir-fry for 3-4 minutes until vegetables are tender-crisp.

- Stir in low-sodium soy sauce and sesame oil, tossing to coat evenly.

- Serve turkey and vegetable stir-fry over cooked brown rice or quinoa.

3. Lentil and Vegetable Soup:

Ingredients:

- 1 cup dried lentils, rinsed
- 1 onion, chopped
- 2 carrots, diced
- 2 celery stalks, diced
- 2 cloves garlic, minced
- 1 teaspoon dried thyme

- 1 teaspoon dried rosemary

- 4 cups low-sodium vegetable or chicken broth

- Salt and pepper to taste

- Fresh parsley, chopped for garnish

Instructions:

- In a large pot, heat olive oil over medium heat. Add chopped onion, diced carrots, and diced celery. Sauté for 5-7 minutes until vegetables begin to soften.

- Add minced garlic, dried thyme, and dried rosemary. Sauté for another 1-2 minutes until fragrant.

- Add rinsed lentils and broth to the pot. Bring to a boil.

- Reduce heat to low, cover, and simmer for 20-25 minutes, or until lentils are tender.

- Season with salt and pepper to taste.
- Serve hot, garnished with fresh chopped parsley.

4. Grilled Salmon with Quinoa and Roasted Vegetables:

Ingredients:

- 2 salmon fillets
- 1 tablespoon olive oil
- Juice of 1 lemon
- Salt and pepper to taste
- 1 cup quinoa, cooked
- Assorted vegetables for roasting (e.g., bell peppers, zucchini, cherry tomatoes)
- Fresh herbs (e.g., thyme, rosemary) for garnish

Instructions:

- Preheat grill to medium-high heat.

- Brush salmon fillets with olive oil and lemon juice. Season with salt and pepper.

- Grill salmon fillets for 4-5 minutes per side, or until fish flakes easily with a fork.

- While salmon is grilling, toss assorted vegetables with olive oil, salt, and pepper. Roast in the oven at 400°F (200°C) for 15-20 minutes, or until vegetables are tender.

- Serve grilled salmon with a side of quinoa and roasted vegetables. Garnish with fresh herbs.

<u>**Tips:**</u>

- **Preparation**: These recipes can often be prepared ahead of time or adapted for meal prepping.

- **Variety**: Experiment with different herbs, spices, and vegetables to customize flavors to your liking.

- **Portion Sizes**: Be mindful of portion sizes to ensure balanced nutrition and avoid overeating.

These dinner recipes provide a range of delicious options that support gallbladder health through nutritious ingredients and cooking methods that are gentle on the digestive system.

Here are some gallbladder-friendly snack and dessert recipes that emphasize wholesome ingredients and are gentle on the digestive system:

Snack Recipes

1. Hummus with Vegetable Sticks:

Ingredients:

- 1 cup chickpeas, drained and rinsed (if using canned)
- 2 tablespoons tahini
- 1 clove garlic, minced
- Juice of 1 lemon
- 2 tablespoons olive oil
- Salt and pepper to taste
- Assorted vegetable sticks (e.g., carrot, cucumber, bell pepper)

Instructions:

- In a food processor, combine chickpeas, tahini, minced garlic, lemon juice, and olive oil.
- Blend until smooth, adding water as needed to reach desired consistency.
- Season with salt and pepper to taste.
- Serve hummus with assorted vegetable sticks for dipping.

2. Greek Yogurt with Berries and Almonds:

Ingredients:

- 1/2 cup plain Greek yogurt
- Handful of fresh berries (e.g., strawberries, blueberries)
- 1 tablespoon sliced almonds

- Drizzle of honey (optional)

Instructions:

- In a bowl, spoon Greek yogurt.
- Top with fresh berries and sliced almonds.
- Drizzle with honey if desired.
- Serve immediately.

Dessert Recipes:

1. Baked Apples with Cinnamon and Walnuts:

Ingredients:

- 2 apples (e.g., Granny Smith or Honeycrisp), cored
- 1 tablespoon maple syrup or honey
- 1/2 teaspoon ground cinnamon
- 2 tablespoons chopped walnuts

Instructions:

- Preheat oven to 375°F (190°C).
- Place cored apples in a baking dish.
- Drizzle maple syrup or honey over apples.
- Sprinkle ground cinnamon and chopped walnuts on top.
- Bake for 20-25 minutes, or until apples are tender.
- Serve warm, optionally with a dollop of Greek yogurt or a sprinkle of granola.

2. Banana-Oat Cookies:

Ingredients:

- 2 ripe bananas, mashed
- 1 cup rolled oats

- 1/4 cup chopped nuts (e.g., almonds, walnuts)
- 1/4 cup raisins or dried cranberries (optional)
- 1/2 teaspoon ground cinnamon
- 1/2 teaspoon vanilla extract
- Pinch of salt

Instructions:

- Preheat oven to 350°F (175°C). Line a baking sheet with parchment paper.
- In a bowl, combine mashed bananas, rolled oats, chopped nuts, raisins or dried cranberries (if using), ground cinnamon, vanilla extract, and a pinch of salt. Mix until well combined.

- Drop spoonfuls of the mixture onto the prepared baking sheet, shaping them into cookies.

- Bake for 15-20 minutes, or until cookies are golden brown and set.

- Remove from oven and let cool on a wire rack.

- Enjoy these healthy cookies as a guilt-free treat!

<u>Tips:</u>

- **Portion Control**: Even with healthier snacks and desserts, moderation is key to maintaining a balanced diet.

- **Customization**: Feel free to adjust these recipes to suit your taste preferences and dietary needs.

- **Hydration**: Enjoy snacks and desserts with a glass of water to stay hydrated throughout the day.

These snack and dessert recipes provide tasty options that support gallbladder health by focusing on nutritious ingredients and minimizing processed sugars and unhealthy fats.

CHAPTER FOUR
Coping With Gallbladder Attacks

Experiencing a gallbladder attack can be distressing and painful. Here are some steps to help cope with and manage gallbladder attacks:

During a Gallbladder Attack:

• **Seek Medical Attention**: If you suspect you're having a gallbladder attack for the first time or if the pain is severe and persistent, seek immediate medical help. Gallbladder attacks can sometimes lead to complications, such as infections or blocked bile ducts, which require medical intervention.

• **Manage Pain**: While waiting for medical assistance or if you have mild symptoms, you can try to alleviate discomfort:

- **Rest**: Lie down and try to relax, as movement can sometimes exacerbate pain.

- **Heat Application**: Applying a heating pad or warm compress to the affected area may help ease pain.

- **Over-the-Counter Pain Relief**: If appropriate and recommended by your healthcare provider, you can take over-the-counter pain medications such as acetaminophen (Tylenol) to help manage pain.

- **Stay Hydrated**: Drink small sips of water if you can tolerate it. Staying hydrated is important for overall health and can help thin bile and ease symptoms.

- **Avoid Solid Foods**: During an attack, it's best to avoid eating solid foods until the pain subsides. This can help reduce the workload on your digestive system and ease discomfort.

<u>After a Gallbladder Attack:</u>

• **Follow Medical Advice**: Once you've received medical attention, follow your doctor's advice regarding further evaluation, treatment options, and any dietary or lifestyle changes you may need to make.

• **Dietary Adjustments**: Your healthcare provider may recommend dietary modifications to prevent future attacks. This often includes reducing intake of fatty or fried foods, increasing fiber intake, and staying hydrated.

• **Monitor Symptoms**: Keep track of your symptoms and any triggers that may have caused the attack. This information can help you and your healthcare provider develop a plan to manage your condition effectively.

• **Consider Surgery (if recommended)**: In some cases, especially if you experience recurrent or severe gallbladder attacks, your doctor may recommend surgical removal of the gallbladder (cholecystectomy) to prevent future complications.

Long-Term Management:

• **Maintain a Healthy Lifestyle**: Adopting a healthy diet, maintaining a healthy weight, and regular physical activity can help support gallbladder health and overall well-being.

• **Stay Informed**: Educate yourself about gallbladder health, symptoms, and preventive measures. This knowledge can empower you to make informed decisions about your health.

• **Regular Follow-Ups**: Attend follow-up appointments with your healthcare provider as recommended to monitor your condition and adjust treatment plans if necessary.

• **Manage Stress**: Stress can sometimes exacerbate digestive issues. Practice stress-reduction techniques such as deep breathing, meditation, or yoga to help manage stress levels.

If you have a history of gallbladder issues or are experiencing symptoms, it's essential to work closely with your healthcare provider to develop a personalized plan for managing and preventing gallbladder attacks.

Post-Surgery Diet Recommendations

After undergoing gallbladder removal surgery (cholecystectomy), it's important to follow dietary recommendations that support healing, aid digestion, and prevent discomfort. Here are some general post-surgery diet recommendations:

Immediate Post-Surgery (First Few Days):

• **Clear Liquids**: Initially, you'll be advised to consume clear liquids such as water, broth, herbal tea, and clear juices. These help prevent dehydration and are easy on the digestive system.

• **Progress to Full Liquids**: As tolerated, you can advance to full liquids like smooth soups, yogurt, and thin porridge. These provide more nutrients while still being gentle on your digestive tract.

Weeks 1-2 Post-Surgery:

• **Low-Fat, Easily Digestible Foods**: Gradually introduce low-fat foods such as:

1. Lean proteins: Skinless poultry, fish, tofu
2. Cooked vegetables: Steamed or lightly sautéed
3. Whole grains: Rice, quinoa, oatmeal
4. Low-fat dairy or dairy alternatives

• **Small, Frequent Meals**: Eat smaller meals throughout the day rather than large meals to reduce stress on your digestive system.

• **Avoid or Limit High-Fat Foods**: Steer clear of fried foods, fatty cuts of meat, creamy sauces, and heavily processed foods. These can be harder to digest and may cause discomfort.

Weeks 3-6 Post-Surgery:

• **Gradually Introduce Fiber**: Begin adding more fiber-rich foods such as fruits (with skins removed), vegetables, whole grains, and legumes. Fiber helps with digestion and bowel regularity.

• **Monitor Tolerance**: Pay attention to how your body reacts to different foods. Some individuals may find certain foods (like spicy or very high-fiber foods) more challenging initially.

<u>Long-Term Dietary Considerations:</u>

• **Balanced Diet**: Aim for a balanced diet that includes a variety of nutrient-dense foods from all food groups: fruits, vegetables, lean proteins, whole grains, and healthy fats.

• **Stay Hydrated**: Drink plenty of water throughout the day to support digestion and overall health.

• **Healthy Eating Habits**: Chew food thoroughly, eat slowly, and avoid eating large meals late at night to aid digestion.

• **Individualized Approach**: Your tolerance for certain foods may vary, so work with your healthcare provider or a dietitian to customize your diet based on your specific needs and preferences.

<u>**Tips for Adjusting to Life Without a Gallbladder:**</u>

• **Moderate Fat Intake**: While you don't need to completely eliminate fats, focus on choosing healthier fats like those found in olive oil, avocados, and nuts.

• **Watch for Symptoms**: Be mindful of any digestive symptoms such as bloating, gas, or diarrhea, especially after eating higher-fat or new foods.

• **Gradual Return to Normal Diet**: Slowly reintroduce foods into your diet to gauge tolerance and prevent discomfort.

By following these post-surgery diet recommendations and making gradual adjustments, you can support your recovery, promote digestion, and maintain overall well-being after gallbladder removal surgery.

CHAPTER FIVE
Lifestyle Tips For Gallbladder Health

Maintaining gallbladder health involves adopting healthy lifestyle habits that support digestion, reduce the risk of gallstones, and promote overall well-being. Here are some essential lifestyle tips for gallbladder health:

• Aim for a healthy weight through a balanced diet and regular physical activity. Obesity is a risk factor for gallstones and gallbladder disease.

• Include plenty of fruits, vegetables, whole grains, lean proteins, and healthy fats in your diet. Limit saturated fats, trans fats, and refined sugars, which can contribute to gallstone formation.

• Drink plenty of water throughout the day. Water helps maintain proper bile production and keeps your digestive system functioning smoothly.

• Fiber helps regulate digestion and may reduce the risk of gallstones. Include fiber-rich foods like fruits, vegetables, whole grains, and legumes in your diet.

• Excessive alcohol intake can contribute to gallbladder problems. If you drink alcohol, do so in moderation.

• Engage in regular physical activity to help maintain a healthy weight, improve digestion, and reduce the risk of gallbladder issues.

• Chronic stress can affect digestion and contribute to digestive disorders. Practice stress management techniques such as deep breathing, meditation, or yoga.

• Rapid weight loss and crash diets can increase the risk of gallstones. Aim for gradual, sustainable weight loss through healthy eating and exercise.

• Maintain regular meal times and avoid skipping meals. This helps regulate bile production and supports digestive health.

• Some medications, particularly hormone-based medications like birth control pills or hormone replacement therapy, may increase the risk of gallstones. Discuss potential risks with your healthcare provider.

• Family history can play a role in gallbladder health. If gallbladder problems run in your family, discuss screening and preventive measures with your healthcare provider.

• Educate yourself about gallbladder health, symptoms of gallbladder issues, and preventive measures. Regular check-ups and screenings can help detect problems early.

By incorporating these lifestyle tips into your daily routine, you can support gallbladder health and reduce the risk of developing gallstones or other gallbladder-related issues. If you have specific concerns or symptoms, consult with your healthcare provider for personalized advice and guidance.

Answering Common Questions About Gallbladder Health

Here are answers to some common questions about gallbladder health:

1. What is the function of the gallbladder?

• The gallbladder stores bile produced by the liver. When you eat, the gallbladder releases bile into the small intestine to help digest fats and aid in the absorption of fat-soluble vitamins.

2. What are gallstones and how do they form?

• Gallstones are hardened deposits of bile components, typically cholesterol or bilirubin, that form in the gallbladder. They can vary in size from tiny grains to large stones. Gallstones form when there is an imbalance in the substances that make up bile, causing them to crystallize and harden.

3. What are the symptoms of gallbladder problems?

<u>**Common symptoms of gallbladder issues include:**</u>

1. Pain in the upper right abdomen or in the center of the abdomen, which can be severe and may radiate to the back or shoulder blades.
2. Nausea and vomiting.
3. Bloating and indigestion.
4. Fever and chills (indicating inflammation or infection).

4. What causes gallbladder problems?

<u>**Several factors can contribute to gallbladder problems:**</u>

1. **Dietary Factors**: High-fat diets, rapid weight loss diets, and diets low in fiber.

2. **Genetics**: Family history of gallstones or gallbladder disease.

3. **Health Conditions**: Conditions like obesity, diabetes, and certain liver diseases.

4. **Gender and Age**: Women, particularly those over 40, are more prone to gallstones.

5. **Medications**: Some medications can increase the risk of gallstones.

5. Can you prevent gallbladder problems?

1. While gallbladder issues cannot always be prevented, you can reduce your risk by:
2. Maintaining a healthy weight through diet and exercise.
3. Eating a balanced diet high in fiber and low in saturated fats.
4. Avoiding rapid weight loss diets.
5. Staying hydrated and limiting alcohol consumption.
6. Managing underlying health conditions.

6. What dietary changes can help support gallbladder health?

To support gallbladder health, consider:

1. Eating a diet rich in fruits, vegetables, whole grains, and lean proteins.
2. Limiting saturated fats, trans fats, and refined sugars.
3. Gradually increasing fiber intake to help regulate digestion.
4. Staying hydrated by drinking plenty of water.

7. What should I do if I suspect I have gallbladder problems?

• If you experience symptoms such as severe abdominal pain, nausea, or vomiting, seek medical attention promptly. Your healthcare provider can evaluate your symptoms, perform diagnostic tests, and recommend appropriate treatment options.

8. Is surgery necessary for gallbladder problems?

• Surgery, specifically cholecystectomy (removal of the gallbladder), is often recommended for gallbladder problems such as recurrent gallstones, inflammation (cholecystitis), or gallbladder disease. It is a common and generally safe procedure that can relieve symptoms and prevent complications.

9. What can I eat after gallbladder removal surgery?

• After gallbladder removal surgery, you may be advised to gradually reintroduce foods into your diet, starting with low-fat, easily digestible options. Examples include lean proteins, cooked vegetables, whole grains, and fruits. It's important to follow your healthcare provider's dietary recommendations for post-surgery recovery.

10. Can I live a normal life without a gallbladder?

• Yes, most people can live a normal, healthy life without a gallbladder. After recovery from surgery, dietary adjustments and lifestyle modifications may be necessary to manage digestion and minimize symptoms, especially related to fat digestion.

Conclusion

Adopting a balanced diet, maintaining a healthy weight, staying hydrated, and being aware of symptoms that may indicate gallbladder issues are all essential components of understanding and caring for your gallbladder health.

By maintaining an active lifestyle, managing stress, and making informed dietary decisions, you can mitigate the risk of gallstones and associated complications and promote digestive health.

Promptly seek medical advice if you are experiencing persistent symptoms or have concerns about your gallbladder's health in order to receive the necessary evaluation and treatment.

With the appropriate attention and care, it is possible to experience a healthy and fulfilling lifestyle and promote gallbladder health.

THE END

www.ingramcontent.com/pod-product-compliance
Lightning Source LLC
Chambersburg PA
CBHW061259250726

48653CB00002B/694